Annil Dhingra
Vipul Sapra
Sahil Rohilla

Working Width In Endodontics

Annil Dhingra
Vipul Sapra
Sahil Rohilla

Working Width In Endodontics

LAP LAMBERT Academic Publishing

Impressum / Imprint

Bibliografische Information der Deutschen Nationalbibliothek: Die Deutsche Nationalbibliothek verzeichnet diese Publikation in der Deutschen Nationalbibliografie; detaillierte bibliografische Daten sind im Internet über http://dnb.d-nb.de abrufbar.

Alle in diesem Buch genannten Marken und Produktnamen unterliegen warenzeichen-, marken- oder patentrechtlichem Schutz bzw. sind Warenzeichen oder eingetragene Warenzeichen der jeweiligen Inhaber. Die Wiedergabe von Marken, Produktnamen, Gebrauchsnamen, Handelsnamen, Warenbezeichnungen u.s.w. in diesem Werk berechtigt auch ohne besondere Kennzeichnung nicht zu der Annahme, dass solche Namen im Sinne der Warenzeichen- und Markenschutzgesetzgebung als frei zu betrachten wären und daher von jedermann benutzt werden dürften.

Bibliographic information published by the Deutsche Nationalbibliothek: The Deutsche Nationalbibliothek lists this publication in the Deutsche Nationalbibliografie; detailed bibliographic data are available in the Internet at http://dnb.d-nb.de.

Any brand names and product names mentioned in this book are subject to trademark, brand or patent protection and are trademarks or registered trademarks of their respective holders. The use of brand names, product names, common names, trade names, product descriptions etc. even without a particular marking in this work is in no way to be construed to mean that such names may be regarded as unrestricted in respect of trademark and brand protection legislation and could thus be used by anyone.

Coverbild / Cover image: www.ingimage.com

Verlag / Publisher:
LAP LAMBERT Academic Publishing
ist ein Imprint der / is a trademark of
OmniScriptum GmbH & Co. KG
Heinrich-Böcking-Str. 6-8, 66121 Saarbrücken, Deutschland / Germany
Email: info@lap-publishing.com

Herstellung: siehe letzte Seite /
Printed at: see last page
ISBN: 978-3-659-68004-5

Copyright © 2015 OmniScriptum GmbH & Co. KG
Alle Rechte vorbehalten. / All rights reserved. Saarbrücken 2015

"Importance of Working width in Endodontics"

Authors

Dr. Dhingra Annil
B.D.S., M.D.S., F.A.G.E., F.I.C.D.
Professor & Head

Dr. Sapra Vipul
B.D.S., M.D.S.
Senior Lecturer

Dr. Rohilla Sahil
B.D.S., M.D.S.

Department of Conservative Dentisrty & Endodontics
D.J College Of Dental Sciences & Research
Modinagar, U.P (India)

Corresponding Address
E-mail: sahilrohila69@gmail.com

TABLES OF CONTENTS

S.No.	CHAPTER	Page No.
1	INTRODUCTION	1
2	DEFINING WORKING WIDTH	3
3	ROOT CANAL ANATOMY- THE CORE OF ENDODONTICS	4
4	SIGNIFICANCE OF WORKING WIDTH	8
5	DETERMINATION OF CORRECT WIDTH FOR CANAL PREPARATION	21
6	ENDODONTIC WORKING WIDTH: CURRENT CONCEPTS AND TECHNIQUES	25
7	FACTORS AFFECTING THE DETERMINATION OF INITIAL WORKING WIDTH AT WORKING LENGTH	28
8	ELIMINATING OR MINIMIZING THE INFLUENCE OF AFFECTING FACTORS	33
9	CURRENT CONCEPTS AND GUIDELINES THE MINIMAL FINAL WORKING WIDTH AT WORKING LENGTH	36
10	SUMMARY	38
11	CONCLUSION	40
12	BIBLIOGRAPHY	42

ANNEXURE I   LIST OF FIGURES
ANNEXURE II   LIST OF TABLES
ANNEXURE III   LIST OF ABBREVIATIONS

ANNEXURE I

LIST OF FIGURES

S. No.	NAME OF FIGURE	PAGE No.
1.	Major Anatomic Components of the Root Canal System	4
2.	Diagrammatic representation of Vertucci's canal configurations	6
3.	Maxillary premolar showing B, Buccal; P, Palatal canals	7
4.	The mesiodistally directed radiograph indicates a flattened distal root canal in a mandibular first molar. In the same tooth, the faciolingual direction of routine radiograph gives an impression of round shaped distal canal.	29
5.	The faciolingual direction of the routine radiograph gives an impression of round shaped canal in a mandibular first premolar. The mesiodistally directed radiograph indicates a flattened root canal in the same tooth.	29
6.	Cross- section of a mandibular first premolar, indicating along oval and irregular root canal. In the same tooth, the faciolingual direction of the routine radiograph may be mistakenly recognized as a round- shaped canal because a mesiodistally directed radiograph is rarely available clinically.	29

ANNEXURE II

LIST OF TABLES

S. No.	NAME OF TABLES	PAGE No.
1.	Suggested preparation size depending on Initial Apical Size	22
2.	Current concepts and guidelines determine the minimal final working width at working length for maxillary teeth	36
3.	Current concepts and guidelines determine the minimal final working width at working length for mandibular teeth	37

ANNEXURE III

LIST OF ABBREVIATION

S. No.	ABBREVIATION	FULL FORM
1	WL	Working Length
2	WW	Working Width
3	MAF	Master Apical File
4	Mx	Maxillary
5	Md	Mandibular
6	ML	Mesiolingual
7	MB	Mesiobuccal
8	et al	Et Alii (And Others)
9	Eg	Exempligratia (For Example)
10	CEJ	Cemento-Enamel Junction
11	K-File	Kerr File
12	H-File	HedstromFile
13	GG	Gates Flidden
14	ANOVA	Analysis of Variance
15	FL	Faciolingual
16	DB	Distobuccal
17	CBCT	Cone Beam Computed Tomography
18	P	Palatal
19	SS	Stainless Steel
20	RDT	Residual Dentin Thickness

21	NiTi	Nickel Titanium
22	Mct	Microcomputed Tomography
23	NaOCl	Sodium Hypochlorite
24	CMI	Canal Master Instrument
25	LS	Light Speed
26	RC	Resin Composite
27	GG	Gates Glidden
28	NIT	Non Instrumentation Technology
29	CT	Computed Tomography
30	ISO	International Organization for Standardization
31	PBS	Phosphate Buffered Saline
32	APS	Apical Preparation Size
33	CHX	Chlorhexidine
34	SEM	Stereo Electron Microscope
35	CT	Computed Tomography
36	PT	Protaper
37	Max	Maximum
38	Min	Minimum
39	IAF	Initial Apical File
40	MAF	Master Apical File
41	CRR	Curvature Radius Ratio
42	Rae	Relative Axis Error
43	Wt	Weight
44	CAD/CAM	Computer Aided Design Computer Aided

		Manufacturing
45	PFM	Porcelain Fused Metal
46	IWW	Initial Working Width
47	FAS	Final Apical Size
48	FWW	Final Working Width
49	CW/CCW	Clockwise/Counter Clockwise
50	GPM	Glide Path Management
51	PTN	ProTaper NEXT
52	TF	Twisted Files
53	GT Files	Greater Taper Files

CHAPTER 1

INTRODUCTION

Root canal shaping is one of the most important steps in canal treatment. It is essential to determine the efficacy of all subsequent procedures, including chemical disinfection and root canal obturation (1) and is the basis for successful endodontic treatment, aiming to debride the root canal (2), to remove contaminated dentin, and to create an ideal canal shape for three-dimensional filling (3). The main objective of a clinician is to mechanically and chemically cleanse the root canal system thoroughly, making it free of microorganisms and their substrates. The canal surface irregularities require proper instrumentation for adequate root canal filling. For this purpose, working length, various cleaning and shaping techniques, and instrument motions have gained importance in endodontics.

The root with a graceful tapering canal and a single apical foramen has long been established as an exception rather than the rule. Bifurcating canals, multiple foramina, fins, deltas, loops, cul-de-sacs, intercanal links, C-shaped canals, and accessory canals have most commonly been faced by the investigators in most teeth (4). Microbes are found in all parts of the root canal system, including fins and anastomoses, and at varying depths (up to 300 µm within the dentinal tubules) (5). However, after instrumentation, they have been reported at less than 34 µm of dentin removal (depending on the type of canal cross section) (6).

The instrumentation of the apical matrix to a large size leads to more anatomical irregularities and increases irrigant exchange in the apical third. Apical enlargement during canal cleaning and shaping procedures increases the likelihood of achieving maximum elimination of bacteria from root canal system (7), though a major part of the canal remains uncleaned even after thorough cleaning and shaping (2). It is very difficult even for the most proficient clinician to predict the exact site and number of root canals present in any tooth before the beginning of the treatment. Even the smallest uncleaned part of the canal significantly affects the success rate of the treatment (4).

Until recently, most investigations have involved counting the number of canals and foramina and categorizing how the canals join or split. Majority of studies have tried to evaluate the shape of the canal systems and its clinical implications than to evaluate the actual preoperative size of the canal (8).

The main aims of instrumentation are as follows:

i. To remove heavily infected dentine from all regions of apical canal wall.
ii. To facilitate placement and replacement of the irrigating solution (9).
iii. To facilitate placement of intracanal medication.
iv. To create an apical stop that facilitates reduced leakage and material extrusion (10).
v. To facilitate obturation procedures.

However, it is recommended not to widen the root canal to a larger extent to avoid unnecessary weakening of the root and increased risk of fracture. Regarding modern concepts, the final canal allows adequate irrigation and close adaptation of the filling material during obturation (11).

Working width (WW) is relatively new concept, which involves perceiving a root canal in both perpendicular (working length) and horizontal (WW) dimensions. Thus, endodontic "working width" has always remained unforgotten dimension during root canal procedure without solid scientific evidence; however, it is still not clear "how large is enough."

CHAPTER 2

DEFINING WORK WIDTH

The concept of working width (WW) was given by Dr. Yi-Tai Jou, Department of Endo, University of Pennsylvania, Philadelphia, PA (12), which is defined as **"the initial and post-instrumentation horizontal dimensions of the root canal system at working length and other levels."** WW is best understood by studying the cross sections of apical canals. If the greater diameter of the original canal is measured, the correct WW is an instrument size slightly bigger than that dimension. It is incorrect to determine the final apical instrument size (master apical file) by measuring the size of constriction. The instrumentation is not aimed to match the size of the final instrumentation with that of the constriction. Smaller size increases the canal diameter by removing hard tissue but barely removing the vital pulp tissue, which causes inflammation of remaining tissues. This concept ignores the fact that most canals enlarge so significantly coronal to the constriction that standard tapered instruments (0.02, 0.04, 0.06, 0.08) are adequate in this region, resulting in underprepared apical canals. It is not always feasible to achieve ideal WW. However, even in such cases, we should try to clean as best as we can.

CHAPTER 3

ROOT CANAL ANATOMY- THE CORE OF ENDODONTICS

The hard tissue surrounding the dental pulp takes a variety of configurations and shapes. A thorough knowledge of tooth morphology, careful interpretation of radiographs, and adequate access and exploration of the tooth's root canal are prerequisites for any root canal treatment. Only after correct completion of this phase of therap , can the clinician perform thorough shaping and cleaning and three-dimensional (3-D) obturation. The correct endodontic result is difficult to obtain if the access is not properly prepared. Practitioners should have a thorough understanding of the internal anatomic relationships of teeth and must be able to visualize these relationships before undertaking the endodontic therapy. Careful evaluation of two or more periapical radiographs, exposed at different horizontal angulations of the x-ray cone, is important to get information about the root canal morphology (12). (Figure 1)

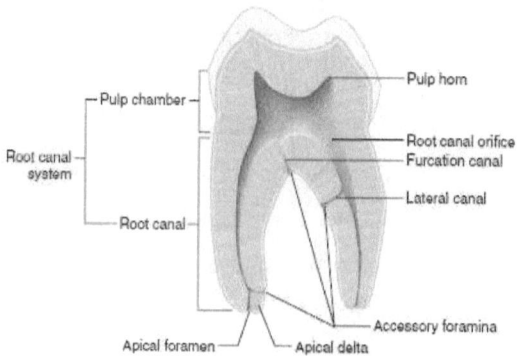

Figure 1: Major Anatomic Components of the Root Canal System

The entire space in the dentin where the pulp is housed is called as the root canal system. The root canal system is divided into two parts : the pulp chamber, that is located in the anatomic crown of the tooth, and the pulp or root canal(s), found in the anatomic root. Other features include the pulp horns;, lateral, accessory, furcation canals; canal orifices; apical deltas; and apical foramina. A root canal begins as a funnel-shaped canal orifice, generally located at or just apical to the cervical line, and ends at the apical foramen (13).

Nearly all the root canals are curved, particularly in a faciolingual direction. These curvatures may create problems during shaping and cleaning procedures because they are not seen on a standard facial radiograph. Different Angled view radiographs are necessary to determine their presence, direction, and severity. A curvature may be a gradual curve of the entire canal or a sharp curvature present near the apex. Double S-shaped canal curvatures also occurs sometimes. In most cases the number of root canals corresponds to the number of roots; but an oval root may have more than one canal (14).

Together with diagnosis and treatment planning, the correct knowledge of common root canal morphology and its frequent variations is a basic requirement for any endodontic success. The significance of canal anatomy has been underscored by different studies demonstrating that variations in canal geometry before shaping and cleaning has a greater impact on the changes that occurred during preparation than did the instrumentation techniques (15).

Weine has categorized the root canal systems in any root into four types., More complex canal system were identified using hematoxylin dye, ; eight pulp space configurations Were Identified , which are as follows:

Type I: A single canal that extends from the pulp chamber to the apex (1).

Type II: Two separate canals leave the pulp chamber and join short of the apex to form the one canal (2-1).

Type III: One canal leaves the pulp chamber and then divides into two in the root; the two then merge to exit as one canal (1-2-1).

Type IV: Two separate, canals extend from the pulp chamber to the apex (2).

Type V: One canal leaves the pulp chamber and divides short of the apex into two separate, distinct canals having separate apical foramina (1-2).

Type VI: Two separate canals leave the pulp chamber, merge in the body of the root, and then redivide short of the apex to exit as two distinct canals (2-1-2).

Type VII: One canal leaves the pulp chamber, divides and then rejoins in the body of the root, and finally redivides into two distinct canals short of the apex (1-2-1-2) (17). (Figure 2)

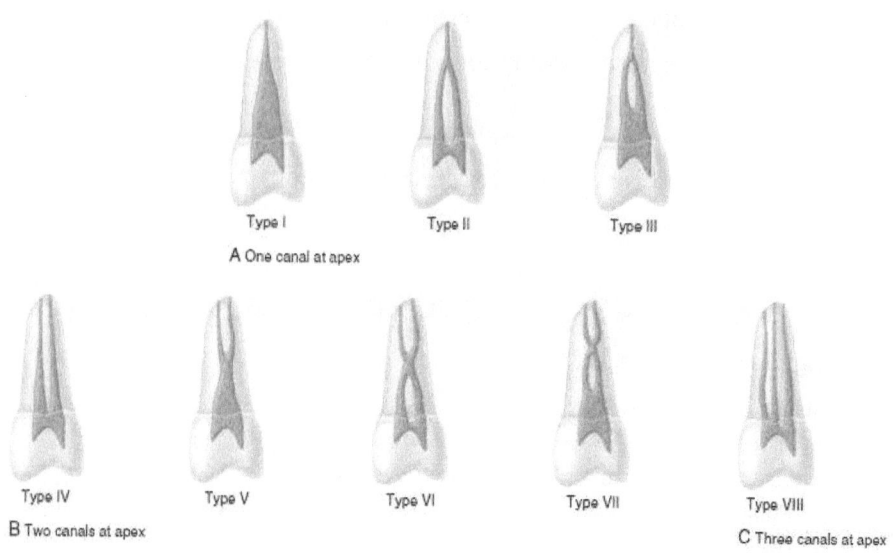

Figure 2: Diagrammatic representation of Vertucci's canal configurations.

The clinician comes across daily with highly complex and variable root canal systems. All available armamentaria should be used to achieve a successful outcome. Proper examination of the pulp chamber floor can reveal clues to the location of orifices and to the type of canal system, If only one canal is present, it is usually located in the center of the access preparation. All such orifices, particularly if oval shaped, must be examined thoroughly with precurved small K-files. If only one orifice is found and is not in the center of the root, then another orifice probably exists, and the clinician should search for it on the opposite side. An oval orifice must be explored with apically curved small instruments. The clinician should place the file tip in the orifice with the tip curved to the buccal side when trying to locate the buccal canal .A curved file tip is placed toward the palate to explore for the palatal canal. Fig 3

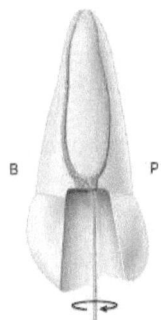

Figure 3: Maxillary premolar showing B, Buccal; P, Palatal canals

CHAPTER 4

SIGNIFICANCE OF WORKING WIDTH

The significance of working width (WW) is as follows:

- ✓ It is required to obtain a round apical stop so as to attain an impermeable seal.

- ✓ It is necessary to determine WW so that the dentinal tubules are microorganism free at the apical 1 mm.

- ✓ Large WW of apical preparation removes more bacteria. It also allows placement of irrigation solutions closer to working length (WL) for easier exchange of irrigants.

Apically shaped canals had significantly reduced bacterial counts in the first session and progressively more so in subsequent instrumentation appointments. It was concluded that irrigants significantly reduced viable bacterial counts (16).

Larger apical preparations help removal of more heavily infected inner dentine to a larger extent. It is also known that irrigants exert a greater antimicrobial effect on superficial dentine than on deep dentine. Canal enlargement will therefore make irrigants accessible to organisms penetrated more deeply into the dentine. Apical enlargement will lead to cleaner apical preparations as measured by the amount of debris remaining (17).

While choosing final apical preparation size, the impact of final canal shape on the root strength should be taken into consideration. Sathorn *et al.* suggested that as the size of rotary NiTi preparations increased, the smoother and rounder canal shape favored elimination of stress concentrations sites, thereby reducing fracture susceptibility (18). Conversely, instruments that lead to irregular dentine removal with canal straightening significantly weaken the root.

Few longitudinal studies have examined the effect of apical enlargement on the outcome of endodontic treatment. Healing was found independent of apical enlargement (19).

Apical preparation is critical in infected root canals and must be directed toward maximizing microbial control. For this, larger apical preparation sizes combined with moderate taper are required (14). In teeth with necrotic infected pulp, bacteria may penetrate to the most apical part of the root canal and have been observed at the apical foramen. Thus, instrumentation length is of utmost importance in infected cases and should presumably not be shorter than the apical level of the root canal up to which bacteria have penetrated (20). Traditionally, the root canal narrows toward the apex to form an apical constriction before expanding to form apical foramen (21). Negishi *et al.* found that teeth in which endodontic instruments were unable to reach the apical foramen had a 5.3 times increased risk of failure than those with an accessible foramen (22).

Schaeffer *et al.* concluded that better healing results are observed in teeth obturated 0–1 mm from the radiographic apex than those obturated more than 1 mm from the apex. However, others have found that the best results are obtained when the root filling extends within 2 mm from the radiographic apex (23). It is confirmed that the apical canal may harbor sufficient microbial load to maintain periapical inflammation, and in light of current evidence, it is recommended that canals should be instrumented and filled to within 0.5 mm of the radiographic apex, unless it is clinically determined that the canal exits at a greater distance.

Orstavik *et al.* (24) and Matsumiya and Kitamura (25) suggested that the size of apical instrumentation may be important for the effective removal of bacteria from the canal. These studies found that with larger instrumentation size maximum bacteria were removed from the canal and the healing was rapid. Kerekes and Tronstad showed that 95% molar mesial canals that they evaluated would have required at least a size 60 apical preparation to fully instrument the apical 1 mm (26).

Inadequate apical cleaning—period— is the reason for the most true endodontic failures. Most important part of the procedure involves proper cleaning and sealing root canals, especially in the apical third. Generally, the instrumentation of the apical third is the most difficult part of the procedure. The narrowest point of the canal is the apical constriction with an average diameter of less than 0.30 mm. However, the canal diameter increases significantly from 0.35 to 1.00 mm coronal to the apical constriction (27).

In general, initial apical canal size has been underestimated. It has been shown that early preflaring improves tactile sensation of the apical constriction and results in more accurate determination of apical diameter.

Hence, if we follow Grossman's criterion of enlarging a root canal to at least three sizes beyond the first file that binds at Working Length (WL), then greater apical enlargement may be needed to ensure that the apical third region is adequately debrided before obturation. Simon considered the apical 3mm of the root canal system to be a "critical" zone in management of infected canals.

Early coronal flaring has been reported to increase the apical file size that binds at working length for both Ni-Ti LS instruments and conventional stainless steel hand files. Early flaring is advantageous, because it shapes the coronal two- third of the canal and removes cervical interference that may provide resistance and affect the operator's ability to pass a file to the apex. Apical preparation is easier when flaring is performed first because only the apical one-third remain unshaped (15).

The initial and post instrumentation horizontal dimensions of the root canal system at working length and other levels are different at different levels in a relatively round canal, the lesser and the greater initial horizontal dimensions are approximately the same.

In an oval, long oval or flat canal, the maximal initial horizontal dimension (MaxIWW) may be several times larger than the minimal initial dimension (MinIWW) at different levels of the canal. For example, in a maxillary cuspid, MinIWW at working length (MinIWW0) may be the same as MaXIWW at working length(MaxIWW0). But 12 mm short of working length, its MaxIWW12 is probably three to four times larger than MinIWW12. This is because at that level, the cross section of a cuspid very often is a long oval or flat canal shape (28).

SIGNIFICANCE OF WORKING WIDTH IN POST AND CORE

- Post is defined as " A custom or proprietary rod that is fitted and cemented into the root canal of an endodontically treated tooth for core retention".

Indications of Post :

Anterior teeth

- Where the natural crown of root-filled teeth either has been lost or is extensively damaged.
- Where the root-filled tooth is to be used as bridge abutment.
- Where a change in axial position greater than 1mm is required.
- Loss of two proximal surfaces with a lingual endodontic access opening which weakens the tooth.

Posterior teeth

- Indicated when the remaining coronal portion is insufficient to support the restoration and sufficient long thick root structure is present.
- Indicated when the root-filled tooth is to be used an abutment for a bridge.
- A shortened tooth – due to the nature of destruction, or removal of undermined, undesirable tooth structure.

Contraindications of Post

1. Severe curvature of the root. Eg: Dilacerations of the root.
2. Persistent periapical lesion
3. Poor periodontal health

4. Poor crown to root ratio
5. Weak / fragile roots
6. Teeth with heavy occlusal contacts
7. Patients with unusual and occupational habits
8. Economic factors
9. Inadequate skill.

CLASSIFICATION OF POSTS

Accoding to INGLE AND BAKLAND

1. Custom cast posts

2. Pre fabricated posts

-Tapered smooth sided

-Parallel sided -

Tapered self -threaded

-Parallel threaded

-Parallel sided with tapered end

ACCODING TO WALTON AND TORABINEJAD

According to shape

1.Parallel

2.Tapered

According to construction

1.Custom made

2.Preformed

According to nature of fit

1.Passive

2.Active

According to surface configuration

1. Smooth

2. Serrated

3. Threaded

ACCORDING TO MATERIALS USED

Metals

1. Custom-cast posts -

Gold alloys -Chrome-cobalt alloys -Nickel-chromium alloys

2. Prefabricated -

Stainless Steel -Titanium

-Brass 3.Non-metals -Carbon-fiber -Fiber-reinforced -Glass fiber -Quartz fiber

-Woven Polyethylene fiber

-Ceramic and zirconia

CUSTOM MADE POSTS

Advantages include:

1. Custom fit to root configuration.
2. Used in large, irregular shaped canals & orifices.
3. Stronger.

Disadvantages include:

1. Higher rate of root fracture.
2. Two appointments.
3. Temporization between appointments.
4. Corrosion can occur due to dissimilar alloys.

PREFABRICATED POSTS

PASSIVE POSTS: TAPERED SMOOTH SIDED

Examples:

-Kerr endopost

-Mooser post

-Ellman Nu bond (*tapered knurled post*)

PASSIVE POSTS: PARALLEL SIDED

Examples:

-Whaledent posts : *parapost*

-Boston post -

Parkell parallel post

-BOSTON POST SYSTEM (*Goldman and Nathanson, Tufts university*)

-99.6% titanium

-Horizontal non engaging serrations

PARKELL PARALLEL POST SYSTEM

-Antirotational lock

-Plastic core formers

-Plastic burn out pattern

PASSIVE POSTS: PARALLEL SIDED WITH TAPERED APICAL ENDS

Examples:

-Degussa

ACTIVE POSTS: SELF THREADING SCREWS

-FLEXIPOST SYSTEM (*tapered*)

-Split shank, parallel sided

ACTIVE POSTS: SELF THREADED

-PARALEL POSTS

Examples:

-Parallel V lock drill and post system

-Parallel Radix Anchor post

ACTIVE POSTS: PARALLEL THREADED POSTS WITH PRE TAPPED CHANNELS

Examples:

-Kurer anchor post

-Pre-tapped, non vented, parallel

NON METALLIC POSTS

-Fiber reinforced posts

-Carbon fiber posts

-Silicon fiber posts

-Woven polyethylene fiber (Ribbond)

Ceramic and zirconium post systems

ADVANTAGES:

1. Esthetics.
2. No corrosion.
3. Extremely biocompatible.
4. Provide improved material strength.

FIBER REINFORCED POSTS

-Carbon fiber posts

-Silicon fiber posts: - S fiber

Glass fiber posts -

Quartz fiber posts

-Woven polethylene fiber : *Ribbond*

CERAMIC AND ZIRCONIA POSTS

Advantages:

1. Translucency and tooth-colored shade.
2. High flexural strength.
3. High fracture resistance.

COMPARATIVE PROPERTIES OF POSTS

According to shape

- Parallel post is retentive than tapered post

According to type

- Active post is better than passive post

According to length

- Long post is retentive than short post

- Intra canal stress patterns in endodontically treated maxillary central incisor having average sized canal diameter and wide canals having three different post systems - cast post and core, carbon fiber post, stainless steel post; that was restored with ceramic crown were recorded. It was concluded that, All the post systems showed maximum stress in the coronal and middle third of the root.
- **Maximum stress was on the inner dentinal wall in the models without reinforcement-**

Stainless steel post > Cast gold > Carbon fiber post.

- **Maximum stress generated in the reinforced model-**

Stainless steel post > Cast gold > Carbon fiber post.

Reinforcement with flowable resin resulted in reduction of stress.

> 3 different types of fiber posts, namely, Carbon fiber posts; Silica-zirconium fiber posts; and Zirconia glass fiber posts; and 3 different types of metal posts namely, Type IV gold cast posts; Stainless steel posts; and Titanium posts were evaluated for flexural modulus and flexural strength in comparison with human root dentin.(29)

- **FLEXURAL MODULUS-**

Dentin Bars < Silica–zirconium fiber posts < Zirconia glass fiber posts < Carbon fiber posts < Gold cast posts < Titanium posts < Stainless steel posts

- **FLEXURAL STRENGTH-**

Dentin Bars < Silica–zirconium fiber posts < Zirconia glass fiber posts < Carbon fiber posts < Titanium posts < Stainless steel posts < Gold cast posts

FRC posts have an elastic modulus that more closely approaches that of dentin while that for metal posts was much higher.

When evaluating the relationship between post form and root fracture, laboratory tests generally indicate that all types of threaded posts produce the greatest potential for root fracture. When comparing tapered and parallel cemented posts using photoelastic stress analysis, the results generally favor the parallel cemented posts. However, the evidence is mixed when the comparison between tapered and parallel posts is based on fracture patterns in extracted teeth created by applying a force via a mechanical testing machine. When evaluating the combined data from multiple clinical studies, threaded posts generally produced the highest root fracture incidence (7%) compared with tapered cemented posts (3%) and parallel cemented (30)

➢ EFFECT OF POST DIAMETER ON RETENTION AND THE POTENTIAL FOR TOOTH FRACTURE

Studies relating post diameter to post retention have failed to establish a definitive relationship. Two studies determined that there was an increase in post retention as the diameter increasedwhereas three studies found no significant retention changes with diameter variations. It was indicated that post length was the most important factor affecting retention and post diameter was a secondary factor. A more definitive relationship has been established between post diameter and stress in the tooth. As the post diameter increased,it was found that stress increases in the tooth .It was found that increasing post diameter decreased the tooth's resistance to fracture. There was a sixfold increase in the potential for root fracture with every millimeter the tooth's diameter was decreased.

- **Post Diameter**

A frequently used and clinically appropriate guideline for post diameter is to not exceed one-third the root diameter. It has been determined that when a root canal is prepared for a post and the diameter is increased beyond one-third of the root diameter, the tooth becomes exponentially weaker. Each millimeter of increase (beyond one-third the root diameter) causes a sixfold increase in the potential for root fracture. The post should be one-third the diameter of root , optimal post diameter measurement should be about 0.6 mm for mandibular incisors and 1.0 mm for maxillary central incisors, maxillary and mandibular canines, and the palatal root of the maxillary first molar. The recommended post diameter for the other teeth was 0.8 mm. Another study of 700 teeth recommended that post diameter should range from 0.7 mm for mandibular incisors.

IMPORTANCE OF DENTIN THICKNESS AFTER ENDODONTIC TREATMENT

Following normal and appropriate endodontic instrumentation, teeth can possess less than 1 mm of dentin, indicating that there should be no further root preparation for the post. When these teeth are encountered, it is best to fabricate a post that fits into the existing

morphologic form and diameter rather than additionally preparing the root to accept a prefabricated type of post. This characteristic is one of the primary indications for use of a **custom cast post and core**. One study determined that canines (maxillary and mandibular), maxillary central and lateral incisors, and the palatal root of maxillary first molars possessed more than 1 mm of dentin after endodontic cleaning and shaping. All other teeth had roots with less than 1 mm of remaining dentin following endodontic treatment. With the goal of preserving 1 mm of remaining dentin lateral to posts, it has been determined that singlecanal maxillary first premolars should have posts that are 0.7 mm in diameter or less. Mandibular premolar having oval- or ribbon-shaped canals should not be subjected to any preparation of the root canal for a post as this will result in less than 1 mm of dentin. Preparation of the mesial root canals in mandibular molars and the buccal root canals in maxillary molars can result in perforation or only thin areas of remaining dentin. Based on measurements of residual dentin thickness, it is recommended that posts not be placed in these roots if possible.

CORE

The restorative materials used to replace missing coronal tooth structure in a root-filled tooth.

IDEAL REQUIREMENTS:

1. Stability in wet environment
2. Rapid, hard set for immediate crown preparation
3. Natural tooth color

4. High compressive strength, tensile strength.

5. High fracture toughness

6. Low plastic deformation

7. Inert (no corrosion)

8. Cariostatic properties

9. Biocompatibility

CORE MATERIALS

-Amalgam

Composite

-Glass ionomer

-Miracle Mix

-Amalgam Core

- **NEWER CORE MATERIALS**

LUXA CORE (DMG)-

- Self curing composite
- Cuts like dentin, very high compressive strength

LUXA CORE Z- DUAL (DMG)-

- Combines DMG-patented nano technology and zirconium dioxide, thus featuring further improved compressive strength and cuttability.

OXFORD ZIRCORE NANO-

KETAC NANO LIGHT-CURING GLASS IONOMER-

- Resin modified glass ionomer indicated for Core build-ups (>50% coronal tooth intact) (31).

CHAPTER 5

DETERMINATION OF CORRECT WIDTH FOR CANAL PREPARATION

At the initial appointment for preparing any canal, the minimum degree of enlargement obtained is of size 20, which allows for the use of a broach for tissue removal in bulk. The smaller size instruments increase the canal diameter by removing hard tissue but merely remove vital pulp tissue, thereby causing inflammation of the remaining tissue (32).

During initial phases of instrumentation, the apical portion of the canal is packed with tissue tags, debris, and other potential irritants. To avoid any chronic inflammation, these need to be removed. So, if enlargement to at least size 20 is not achievable for a canal at any given appointment, it is best not to perform any enlargement on the canal, for example, in the treatment of mandibular molar with vital pulp.

If the first appointment allows for only access preparation, pulpotomy, and enlargement of large canal, it is better to leave the smaller canals untouched. Even determining working length (WL) using radiographic methods should be avoided. At the next appointment, the smaller canals are enlarged to a minimum of size 20 and allowed for broaching of the entire canal length.

The apical width is determined by first recognizing the initial apical file (IAF), which is the first size of the file binding at full WL (Table 1). Using circumferential filing motion, the canal is then enlarged to three full sizes larger than this initial file, which is called the master apical file (MAF).

Chapter 5- Determination of Correct width for Canal Preparation

Table 1: Suggested preparation size depending on Initial Apical Size

Initial file that binds	Area at D1 (sq mm)	Probable MAF	Area at D1 (Sq mm)	Final Flare Size
10	0.00785	25 or 30	0.0491	40 or 45
15	0.01766	30	0.0707	45
20	0.0314	35	0.0962	50
25	0.0491	40	0.1256	55
30	0.0707	45	0.1590	60
35	0.0962	50	0.1963	70
40	0.1256	55	0.2375	80

Enlargement in Moderately Wide and Straight Canals

Typical canals involved in this type of preparation are maxillary anteriors, wider one-canalled mandibular cuspids and bicuspids, one-canalled maxillary bicuspids, and largest molar canals. These canals will accommodate a size 25 or larger IAF and size 40 or larger MAF.

Traditional method of preparation

After calculating the WL, it is made sure that IAF is loose before going to the next larger size. The canal is enlarged to proper MAF through proper rasping and circumferential filing. The file one size larger than the MAF is selected and the canal is enlarged at the level of 1-mm short of the WL. Go back to the full WL with the MAF. Then, the larger files are selected progressively and canal is enlarged at the level of 2- and 3-mm short of the WL. Go back to the full WL with the MAF at each progressive step.

Technique used with non-ISO tapered files

The WL is calculated and IAF is selected and made loose using rasping motion. A large size 0.04 non-ISO tapered file is selected with a stop at the WL minus 2 mm, not going beyond the length indicated by the stop. The IAF is then passed to the WL using rasping action. The next larger size 0.04 non-ISO tapered file is selected with the stopper at the same length and canal is filed down toward the apex. Step 3 is then repeated. Then, a file one size larger than the IAF is used and the preparation up through the MAF is continued.

Enlargement in Smaller, Relatively Straight Canals

For this type of preparation, typical canals include mandibular incisors, bicanalled mandibular cuspids, bicanalled maxillary bicuspids, and smaller molar canals.

Technique

The canal is slowly enlarged with the IAF. Incremental instrumentation is used and clip 1 mm off the tip of the file using Glyde or NaOCl as the irrigant. An intermediate size 0.04 tapered file is selected with a stopper at the WL minus 2 mm and file toward the apex. The IAF is passed to the WL using a rasping motion. The next larger size 0.04 non-ISO tapered file is selected with the stopper at the same length and canal is filed down toward the apex. Step 3 is then repeated. The next large size 0.04 non-ISO tapered file is selected with the stopper at the same length and canal is filed down toward the apex. Again a file one size larger than the IAF is used, and the preparation up through the MAF is continued.

Importance of Using MAF as Final Instrument after Using Flaring Files Short of the Working Length

Failure to use the MAF as the last file (at WL) in the canal can lead to major errors in small curved canals. Use of the wider flaring files short of the WL may leave small ledges in the canal and may pack dentinal filings toward the apex. To obtain a smooth passage for the gutta-percha at the full WL, it is better to use the MAF in the end.

Wu et al. (10) conducted a study to determine whether the first file that binds at the WL corresponds to the canal diameter. They concluded that neither the first K-file nor the first Light Speed instrument to bind reflected the canal diameter at the WL. As a result, canal preparation three sizes larger than this file does not assure removal of inner layer of dentine from of the entire canal wall. Thus, using the first file to bind for gauging the diameter of the apical canal and as guidance for apical enlargement is not reliable (33).

CHAPTER 6

ENDODONTIC WORKING WIDTH: CURRENT CONCEPTS & TECHNIQUES

MinIWW(N)	Minimal initial horizontal dimension N-mm short of working length (WL)
MinIWW0	Minimal initial horizontal dimension at WL
MinIWW1	Minimal initial horizontal dimension 1-mm short of WL
MinIWW2	Minimal initial horizontal dimension 2-mm short of WL
MaxIWW(N)	Maximal initial horizontal dimension N-mm short of WL
MaxIWW0	Maximal initial horizontal dimension at WL
MaxIWW1	Maximal initial horizontal dimension 1-mm short of WL
MaxIWW2	Maximal initial horizontal dimension 2-mm short of WL
MinFWW(N)	Minimal final horizontal dimension N-mm short of WL
MinFWW0	Minimal final horizontal dimension at WL
MinFWW1	Minimal final horizontal dimension 1-mm short of WL
MinFWW2	Minimal final horizontal dimension 2-mm short of WL
MaxFWW(N)	Maximal final horizontal dimension N-mm short of WL
MaxFWW0	Maximal final horizontal dimension at WL
MaxFWW1	Maximal final horizontal dimension 1-mm short of WL
MaxFWW2	Maximal final horizontal dimension 2-mm short of WL

In a relatively round canal, MinIWW and MaxIWW are approximately the same. In an oval, long oval, or flat canal, MaxIWW is several times larger than MinIWW at different levels of the canal.

In a maxillary cuspid (before instrumentation), $MinIWW0$ may be the same as $MaxIWW0$, whereas $MaxIWW12$ may be three to four times larger than $MinIWW12$. On the other hand, after instrumentation, $MinFWW0$ may the same as $MaxFWW0$ (considering no significant transportation). However, the ratio between $MinFWW12$ and $MaxFWW12$ may be altered by mechanical preparation of the canal.

Current Descriptions of the Horizontal Dimensions (Cross Sections) of the Root Canal

1. *Round (circular) canal*: MaxIWW equals MinIWW.

2. *Oval canal*: MaxIWW is greater than MinIWW (up to two times more).

3. *Long oval canal*: MaxIWW is two or more times greater than MinIWW (up to four times more).

4. *Flattened (flat, ribbon) canal*: MaxIWW is four or more times greater than MinIWW.

5. *Irregular canal*: It cannot be defined by list points 1–4 (12).

Determination of Initial Working Width at Working Length

1. First determine the preoperative canal diameter by passing consecutively larger instruments to the WL until one binds. This initial apical file estimation is referred to as the determination of $MinIWW0$.

2. Then, the master apical file size ($MaxFWW0$) is suggested to be three ISO file sizes larger than that initial binding file.

But this concept is being questioned as recent studies suggest that the first k file that binds at the WL did not accurately reflect the diameter of the apical canal. The inaccuracy and discrepancy is the result of various morphologic and procedural factors as each of the factor discussed further can affect the clinician's tactile sense.

CHAPTER 7

FACTORS AFFECTING THE DETERMINATION OF WORKING WIDTH AT WORKING LENGTH

Canal Morphology

Canal morphology is a critically important part of root canal therapy. Various *in vitro* studies have recorded the scales and average sizes of root canals (14), but only few clinical attempts have been made to determine the working width (WW). Sectioning of all levels of the teeth and making section plane exactly perpendicular to the canal curvature is a difficult task. Therefore, most morphometric studies cannot exactly depict the horizontal dimensions of root canal system. Until recently, most investigations have involved counting the number of canals and foramina and categorizing the canals based on the manner in which they join or split.

Current studies focus more on the shape of the canal systems and its clinical implications than on the actual, preoperative size of the canal (8). The horizontal dimension of the root canal system is not only more complicated than the vertical dimension but also more difficult to investigate because it varies greatly at each vertical level of the canal as shown in Figs. 6.1–6.3. The round canal can be measured more easily because the minimum initial working width (MinIWW) and maximum initial working width are the same. However, other factors make initial working width (IWW) determination difficult, even in straight canals. To determine the MinIWW of the oval, long oval, and flat canals, we may need proper instrument and tactile sensation.

The presence of undetected lingual canal or an untreated isthmus may be responsible for endodontic failure of lower incisors. The prevalence of two canals in mandibular incisors has been has been found to be 11.5%–44.1%, although many merge into single canal in the apical 1–3 mm of the root.

Sectioning of root is the most common method for evaluating the shape of the canal. Cross sections at different levels in a root allow direct viewing of canal shape and position with regard to the borders of the root surface (figure 4-6) (17).

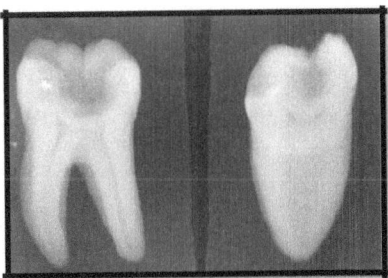

Fig 4. The mesiodistally directed radiograph indicates a flattened distal root canal in a mandibular first molar. In the same tooth, the faciolingual direction of routine radiograph gives an impression of round distal canal.

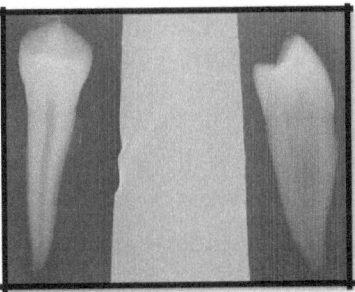

Fig 5. The faciolingual direction of the routine radiograph gives an impression of round canal in a mandibular first premolar. The mesiodistally directed radiograph indicates a flattened root canal in the same tooth.

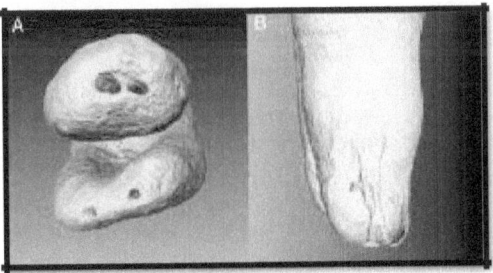

Fig 6. Cross- section of a mandibular first premolar, indicating along oval and irregular root canal. In the same tooth, the faciolingual direction of the routine radiograph may be mistakenly recognized as a round canal because a mesiodistally directed radiograph is rarely available clinically.

Canal length

When using an instrument to measure working length (WL), the longer the canal, the higher the friction resistance. In a very long canal (>25 mm), the friction resistance may increase to affect the tactile sense of the clinician to determine the IWW correctly. In addition, if the coronal flare is too conservative or limited to the coronal third of the canal, then shaft of the instrument may engage the canal wall and lead to a false/premature conclusion regarding WW.

Canal taper

Any discrepancy between the gauging instrument and canal due to tapering can cause an early engagement of the canal wall with the instrument, leading to a false sensation of apical binding. The tapering of the canal may increase due to early coronal flare; however, the tapering discrepancy between the gauging instrument and canal wall may decrease. The last 3–5 mm of the canal has parallel walls, making accurate determination of IWW. The root canal content may be fibrous or calcified material (calcific metamorphosis) creating different degrees of frictional resistance against the gauging instrument. This eventually affects the tactile sense of the clinician to determine the IWW accurately.

Canal curvature

Curved canals can deflect the gauging instrument and increase friction resistance. The root canal curvature can be categorized as two dimensional, three dimensional, with small radius, with large radius, and double curvature (S- shaped, Bayonet shaped), and with different degrees of severity. Each of these curvatures has a different effect on the tactile sense of a clinician. The combination of these curvatures makes determination of IWW a difficult task, if not possible. The study by Wu *et al.* (10) indicated that in curved mandibular premolars, the first K-file and the first Light Speed instrument that bound at the WL failed to accurately reflect the diameter of the apical canal (10).

Success of the root canal therapy depends on careful canal preparation. The main aim of endodontic instrumentation is to enlarge a canal without deviating from the original canal curvature.

It has been stated that "The final preparation should be an exact replica of the original canal configuration in shape, taper and flow, only larger."

Canal curvature

Curved canals can cause deflection of the gauging instrument and increase friction resistance. The curvature of the root canal can be categorized into two dimensional, three dimensional, small radius, large radius, and double curvature (S-shaped, Bayonet shaped) and with different degree of severity. Each of these curvatures has a different effect on a clinician's tactile sense. The combination of these curvatures make correct determination of Initial Working Width extremely difficult, if not possible. In curved mandibular premolars, the study by Wu et al indicated that the first K file and the first Light speed instrument that bound at the Working Length failed to accurately reflect the diameter of the apical canal. (10).

Careful canal preparation is an important part of successful root canal therapy. The ability to enlarge a canal without deviation from the original canal curvature is a primary objective in endodontic instrumentation. It has been stated that "The final preparation should be an exact replica of the original canal configuration in shape, taper and flow, only larger". After studying the effects of several instrumentation techniques, it is noted that every file, whether precurved or straight, tended to straighten within the canal (13). They reported that the largest amount of apical canal preparation occurred at the outer portion of curvature, away from the furcation.

An attempt to solve this problems has led to the development of various instrumentation technique like step back, crown down, balanced force, anti curvature filling etc in addition several instruments like K flex, flex arc, flex- o, Protaper, race files, light speed, hero shaper-hands and rotary files have been designed. This instruments aim at alleviating procedural difficulties at coronal, middle, apical regions of root canal. The Schneider method is the primary technique used to measure canal angulation.

Canal wall irregularities

Attached pulp stones, denticles and reparative dentin can create convexities on the canal wall surface. Resorption can produce concavities on the canal wall surface. These phenomena can serve as an impacting factor that induces a false estimation of the true canal dimension at working length and other levels.

Instrument for determining initial working width

The rigidity and tapering of the instrument used for determining IWW can affect accuracy. Any tapering discrepancy between the gauging instrument and canal may lead to an early instrument engagement of the canal wall, altering the tactile sensation. The rigid instrument in a curved canal also lead to a false tactility.

CHAPTER 8

ELIMINATING THE INFLUENCE OF AFFECTING FACTORS

Prior to determining the initial working width (IWW), the orifices should be widened for early coronal flaring (crown down, double flaring), which ensures effective irrigation and minimizes any interferences with tactile sensation. To avoid interference and to achieve better results, an adequate instrument with maximal flexibility and minimal taper should be used. The exact outline of the horizontal dimensions of the root canal should be followed by root canal preparation at every level of the canal. To minimize incomplete cleaning of the root canal system, circumferential preparation or instrumentation need to be taken into consideration. A continuous reaming action of most of the nickel–titanium (NiTi) rotary instruments makes the canal relatively circular. Incomplete cleaning of the root canal system may be a result of imprudent use of the NiTi rotary instruments alone, which leads to failure of the endodontic therapy.

Determination of the Minimal and Maximal Final Working Width at Working Length

A final working width is required for bacteria and their substrates removal, and also for dead pulp tissue removal. Further, it is necessary to increase the capacity of the root canal to retain a larger amount of sterilizing agent and also to prepare the tooth to receive the canal filling (12).

To increase the success rate of the treatment, it is essential to remove the infected dentin. For this purpose, the instruments and techniques used should help in retaining the original shape of the canal to maximize the cleaning effectiveness and minimize unnecessary weakening of tooth structure.

Chapter 8 - Eliminating the Influence of Affecting Factors

How Do We Know When the Final Apical Instrument Size Is Reached?

By instrumenting and cross sectioning many teeth, it has been concluded that no technique is perfect, and a correct WW is a clinical judgment. However, instrument that meets resistance 4–5 mm short of working length (WL) and then requires a firm push to reach WL closely approximates the correct WW.

The instrument that approximates the correct WW the final apical size. Rotary system has been found to be very important for achieving larger apical preparations safely. In its original form (stainless steel and hand driven), NiTi rotary system evolved through the 1990s and 2000s from improvements made to the earlier versions.

Majority of rotary systems comprise a very short cutting blade, a non-cutting pilot tip, and a smooth flexible taperless shaft.

This provides it maximum flexibility to negotiate curves and cut dentin from canal walls, maintaining canal anatomy without the need for excessive mid-root or coronal over enlargement. Because only the very tip of the instrument comes in contact with canal walls, the tactile sensation is incomparable. Rotary system is extremely safe because of its safety release feature that aids the instrument to separate at the handle instead of at the tip when excessive twisting forces are encountered.

HOW DO WE KNOW WHEN THE FINAL APICAL INSTRUMENT SIZE IS REACHED?

By instrumenting and the cross- sectioniong many teeth it has been concluded that no technique is perfect, and a correct working width is a clinical judgement. However, instrument that meets resistance 4 to 5 mm short of working length and then requires a firm push to reach working length closely approximates the correct working width. The instrument that approximates the correct working width the Final Apical Size (FAS). To achieve larger apical preparations, safely, Rotary system has been found to be invaluable. In its original form (stainless steel and hand driven), NiTi rotary system, evolved through the 1990s and 2000s from improvements made to earlier versions.

Majority of rotary systems have :

- ✓ A very short cutting blade
- ✓ A non-cutting pilot tip
- ✓ A smooth flexible taperless shaft.

This affords it maximum flexibility to negotiate curves and cut dentin from canal walls maintaining canal anatomy without the need for excessive mid- root or coronal over enlargement. Tactile feel is unequalled because only the very tip of the instrument comes in contact with canal walls. Rotary system is extremely safe due to its safety release feature which causes the instrument to separate at the handle instead of at the tip when excessive twisting forces are encountered.

CHAPTER 9

CURRENT CONCEPTS AND GUIDELINES DETERMINE THE FINAL WORKING WIDTH AT WORKING LENGTH

Table 2. Maxillary Teeth

Tooth	Grossman	Tronstad	Glickman	Weine
Maxillary centrals	80-90	70-90	35-60	3 Sizes
Maxillary laterals	70-80	60-80	25-40	3 Sizes
Maxillary canines	60-90	50-70	30-50	3 Sizes
Maxillary first premolar	30-40	35-90	24-40	3 Sizes
Maxillary second premolar	50-55	35-90	25-40	3 Sizes
Molars	30-55-50			3 Sizes
Mesiobuccal/distobuccal	35-60	25-40		3 Sizes
Palatal	80-100	25-50		3 Sizes

TABLE 3

Mandibular Teeth

Tooth	Grossman	Tronstad	Glickman	Weine
Mandibular Centrals	40-50	35-70	25-40	3 Sizes
Mandibular Laterals	40-50	35-70	25-40	3 Sizes
Mandibular Canines	50-55	50-70	30-50	3 Sizes
Mandibular First Premolars	30-40	35-70	30-50	3 Sizes
Mandibular Second Premolars	50-55	35-70	30-50	3 Sizes
Mandibular Molars	30-55-50			3 Sizes
Mb/Ml	35-45	25-40		3 Sizes
D	40-80	25-50		3 sizes

CHAPTER 10

SUMMARY

For successful root canal preparation using rotary instruments, careful reviewing of the specific anatomy of each case is extremely important. Straight access should be created into the root canal middle third, with extended access cavities and early coronal flaring. Extra care is required when using rotary instruments in canals that are curved, recurved, dilacerated, divided, or merged. Early coronal enlargement to the same extent as in the case of regular canals is not feasible in very long narrow canals, which results in an increased frictional contact area and the potential for torsional overloading. No ideal solution exists to this problem, except for being extra careful while flaring and potentially using hand instruments (34).

Bends with a small radius of curvature (also called acute bends), more coronally put an instrument with larger cross section under cyclic fatigue and may cause breakage (35). Here coronal flaring to the point of curvature and the use of less-tapered rotary files to the working length (WL) are indicated. Ovoid canals that are wide in buccolingual dimension, such as distal canals of mandibular molars or some premolars, face a different problem. Instrument fracture is unlikely, but they can rarely be prepared to be round, hence debridement may be incomplete. It may be appropriate to approach these cases as if two canals existed buccally and lingually, and then merge preparations by filling action using ultrasonic or hand files.

Preparation of a straighter canal to WL and the other canal to the merging point is recommended for merging canals. This prevents forcing a rotary instrument through a sharp S-shaped curve. For acute curves and narrow canals various procedures have been suggested, although none is certain to be universally successful.

Irrigation is commonly applied using a syringe and a needle, with needle sizes varying typically between 27 and 30 gauge, respectively. With such a system, irrigation solution will not travel apically more than 1 mm beyond the tip of the needle. Thus, it is desirable to place the irrigation solution into periapical tissues. Serious incidents have been reported after NaOCl expressed into maxillary sinus or close to nerves.

With careful use, the benefits of deep intracanal irrigation clearly seem to outweigh the risks.

In fact, the closeness of the irrigation needle to the apex is very important for root canal debris removal. Druttman and Stock found that irrigation performance varied with the size of the needle and the volume of the irrigant, whereas Walton and Torabinejad stated that perhaps the most important factor is the delivery system and not the irrigating solution.

Canal size and shape are very important to the penetration of the irrigant. The apical 5 mm of the canal is not flushed with the irrigant until it has size 30 and more often size 40 file. Needles with small diameters were found to be more effective in reaching adequate depth but have problems such as possible breakage and difficulty in expressing the irrigant from the narrow needles (36).

Recently, Hsieh *et al.* compared a shaped root canal to a "wind tunnel" and evaluated the behavior of irrigation solutions deposited into various depths of flared canals from irrigation needles measuring from 23 to 27 gauge.

A disturbed laminar flow of irrigants was found to be present with a combination of sufficiently enlarged canals, deep needle insertion, and small needle diameter, for example, a 27-gauge needle placed 3 mm from the apex in a canal prepared to size 30 (37).

CHAPTER 11

CONCLUSION

The importance of the horizontal dimensions or working width (WW) of the root canal system has not been addressed in most of the research. In long oval or flat canal preparations, the WW is very important as it alters the operator to the possibilities of incomplete root canal preparation. The concepts, techniques, and technologies to measure initial horizontal dimensions and to determine final horizontal dimensions accurately or properly are underdeveloped.

Understanding the current concepts and techniques of cleaning and shaping of root canal system; carefully maintaining the aseptic chain, using adequate irrigating solutions to enhance efficacy; and cautiously applying current concepts and techniques of WW may provide a better quality of endodontic therapy for the patient.

In vitro studies found manual circumferential filing to be statistically significantly effective than rotary instrumentation for cleaning flattened root canals. The concept of the WW indicated that different approaches and techniques are needed to improve root canal preparation and promote better quality of root canal treatment (38).

Because we cannot see deep into curved canals, we rely on an instrument tactile feedback to provide clue about canal anatomy. Canal statistics are easily available, but because canals differ widely we are working blindly without feedback.

Let us stop thinking canals to be basically of the same size and shape because they are not. The solution is to stop guessing and begin using instruments that provide accurate feedback. We should customize every one of our canal preparations (39).

Treating canals similarly is like forcing everyone to wear the same size shoe-one size doesn't fill all!

—Spanberg

Respect the canal morphology diameter variability as the fingerprint of a person, which is never similar.

—Shashin J Shah

CHAPTER 12

BIBLIOGRAPHY

1. Anil Dhingra, Rohit Kochar, Satyabrat Banerjee, Punit Srivastava. Comparative Evaluation Of The Canal Curavature Modifications After Instrumentation With One Shape Rotary And Wave One Reciprocating Files. JCD 2014, 17:2 ;138-141

2. Anant Patil , Shalini Aggarwal. To Compare and Contrast Maintenance of Root Canal Geomerty Using Rotary NiTi Syatems- An In vitro Study. medind.nic.in/eaa/t13/i1/eaat13i1p14.pdf

3. Nitin Maintin, Arunagiri D, Dexter Brave, Shipra Nangalia Maitin, Sandeep Kaushik, Saumya Roy. JCD 2013, 16:3; 219-223.

4. A.P Tikku, W.Pragya Pandey, Ivy Shukla. Intricate Internal Anantomy of Teeth and Its Clinical Significance In Endodontics –A Review. medin.nic.in/eaa/t12/i2/eaat12i2p160.pdf

5. L.G Coldero, S McHugh, D MacKenzie & W.P. Saunders. Reduction In Intracanal Bacteria During Root Canal Preparation With And Without Apical Enlargement. IEJ 2002, 35, 437-446.

6. Frank Paque, Marc Balmer, Thomas Attin, Ove A. Peters. Preparation Of Oval-Shaped Root Canals In Mandibular molars Using Nickel- Titanium Rotary Instruments: A Micro- Computed Tomography Study. JOE 2010, 36:4; 703-705

7. Siquera JF Jr, Lima KC, M Agalhaes F Ac, Lopes HP, De Uzeda M . Mechanical Reduction of Bacterial Population In Root Canal By Three Instrumentation Technique. JOE 1999,25; 332-335

8. Mauger MJ, Schindler WG, Walker WA. An Evalution Of Canal Morphology At Different Levels Of Root Resection IN Mandibular Incisors. JOE 1998, 24:10; 607-609

9. Wu M, Wesselink PR. Efficacy of Three Techniques In Cleaning The Apical Portion Of Curved Canals. Oral Surgery, Oral Medicine and Oral Pathology 1995, 79; 492-496

10. Wu Mk, Barkis D, Rosis A, Wesselink PR .Does The First File To Bind Correspond To The Diameter Of The Canal In The Apical Region ? IEJ 2002, 35:3;264-266

11. Lars Bergmans, John Van Cleynenbreugel, Marine Wevers, & Paul Lambrechts. Mechanical Root Canal Preparation With NiTi Rotary Instruments: Rationale, Performance And Safety.American Journal Of Dentistry 2001, 14:5; 324-332

12. Friedman S, Moshonov J, Stabholz A: Five root canals in a mandibular first molar. Dent Traumatol 2:226, 1986.

13. Burch JG, Hulen S: The relationship of the apical foramen to the anatomic apex of the tooth root. Oral Surg Oral Med Oral Pathol 34(2):262, 1972.

14. Vertucci FJ: Root canal anatomy of the human permanent teeth. Oral Surg Oral Med Oral Pathol 58:589, 1984.

15. Hata G, Hayami S, Weine FS, Toda T: Effectiveness of oxidative potential water as a root canal irrigant. Int Endod J 34:308, 2001.

16. Vertucci FJ, Seelig A, Gillis R: Root canal morphology of the human maxillary second premolar. Oral Surg Oral Med Oral Pathol 38:456, 1974.

17. Yi-Tai Jou, Bekir Karabucak, Jeffrey Levin, Donald Liu. Endodontic Working Width : Current Concepts And Techniques. Dent Clin N Am 2004, 48; 323-335 18. Tapish Garg, Meenu Garg .Working Width-The Forgotten Dimension. IJRID 2013, 3:4; 64-70

19. GR Young, P Parashos, H H Messer.The Principles of Techniques For Cleaning Root Canals. Australian Dental Journal Supplement 2007, 52 :1Supp ; S52-S63

20. Sathom C, Palamara JEA, Messer HH. Effect Of Root Canal Size And External Root Surface Morphology On Fracture Susceptibility And Pattern: A Finite Element Analysis. J.Endod 2005; 31:288-292

21. Kerekes K. Evaluation Of Standardized Root Canal Instruments And Obturating Points. J Endodon 1979, 5;145-150

22. Wu MK, Fan B, Wessenlink P. Leakage Along Apical Root Filling In Curved Canals. Part I: Effect Of Apical Tranportation On Seal Of Root Filling. J Endodon 2000,26;210-216

23. Yury Kuttler. Microscopic Investigation Of Root Apexes. Journal Of American Dental Association 1955,50 ;544-560

24. Negishi J, Kawanami m, Ogami E. Risk Ananlysis Of Failure Of Root Canal Treatment For Teeth With Inaccessible Apical Constriction. J Dent 2005, 33:399-404

25. A comparative study of intra canal stress pattern in endodontically treated teeth with average sized canal diameter and reinforced wide canals with three different post systems using finite element analysis. Kaur A, Meena N, Shubhashini N, Kumari A, Shetty A. J Conserv Dent 2010;13:28-33)

26. Resistance to fracture of endodontically treated teeth restored with different post systems. Begüm Akkayan, Dr Med Dent, and Turgut Gülmez. J Prosthet Dent 2002; 87:431-7.

27. Restoration of endodontically treated teeth: A guide for the restorative dentist. Charles T. Smith/Nortnan Schuman. Quintessence Int 1997:28:457-462

28. Michelle A. Schaeffer, Robert R. White And Richard E. Walton. Determinig The Optimal Obturation Length: A Meta-Analysis Of Literature. JOE 2005,31:4;271-274

29. Orstavik D, Kerekes K, Molven O. Effects of extensive apical reaming and calcium hydroxide dressing on bacterial infection during treatment of apical periodontitis:a pilot study. Int Endod J 1991, 24;1-7

30. Matsumiya S, Kitamura M. Histo-pathological and histo-bacteriological studies of the relationship between the condition of sterilization of the interior of the root canal and the healing process of periapical tissues in experimentally infected root canal treatment. Bull Tokoyo Dent Coll 1960,1;1-7

31. Kerekes K, Tronstad L. Morphometeric Observation In Root Canals Of Human Premolars. J Endod 1997,3;74

32. Tapish Garg, Meenu Garg. Working Width – The Forgotten Dimension. IJRID 2013.3:4; 64-70

33. E. Steve Senia . Endoodntic Success: It's All About The Apical Third. Endo Tribune 2008, 8-11

34. Schilder H. Cleaning And Shaping The Root Canal . Dent Clin North Am 1974,18;269-296

35. Franklin S.Weine. Endodontic Therapy 6th Edition.1167-1179

36. Shashin J.Shah, Jayshree S. Shah. Wonderful World of Endodontic Working Width – The Forgotten Dimension –A Review. Journal Of Dental Sciences 2005, 2:2;20-26

37. Ruddle C. Cleaning and shaping of root canal system. In: Cohen S, Burns RC, editors. Pathways of the pulp. 8th ed. St. Louis, MO: Mosby; 2002.p.231

38. Pruett JP, Clement DJ, Carnes DL. Cyclic Fatigue testing of nickel- titanium endodontic instruments. J Endod 1997;23:77

39. Chow TW. Mechanical effectiveness Of Root Canal Irrigation. J Endod 1983;9:475

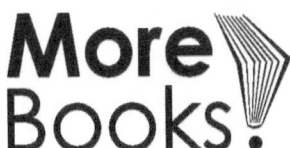
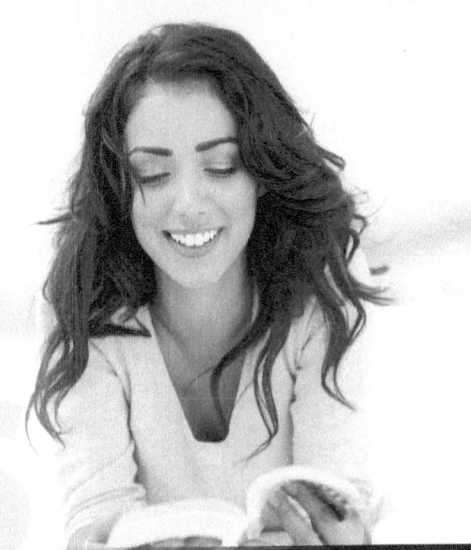

I want morebooks!

Buy your books fast and straightforward online - at one of the world's fastest growing online book stores! Environmentally sound due to Print-on-Demand technologies.

Buy your books online at
www.get-morebooks.com

Kaufen Sie Ihre Bücher schnell und unkompliziert online – auf einer der am schnellsten wachsenden Buchhandelsplattformen weltweit!
Dank Print-On-Demand umwelt- und ressourcenschonend produziert.

Bücher schneller online kaufen
www.morebooks.de

OmniScriptum Marketing DEU GmbH
Heinrich-Böcking-Str. 6-8
D - 66121 Saarbrücken
Telefax: +49 681 93 81 567-9

info@omniscriptum.com
www.omniscriptum.com

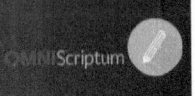

www.ingramcontent.com/pod-product-compliance
Lightning Source LLC
Chambersburg PA
CBHW031549210526
45464CB00003B/1219